UNBREAKABLE, BUT NOT INVINCIBLE!

STORIES OF SURVIVAL...

BY
SCOTT FRASER

I'm writing this memoir in honor of my stepdaughter, Chelsea Lewis.

INTRODUCTION

This book is written in loving memory of Chelsea Lewis...Bright, kind, and full of promise.

Chelsea had just graduated high school and was preparing for the next chapter of her life at University when, in an instant, she was taken from us. That early morning, August 7th, 2022, changed our lives forever, especially for her Mother, Tanja, who lost her only child...it was heartbreaking beyond words.

Chelsea didn't get a second chance, and that truth stayed with me. As her stepfather, I've often reflected on life where fate could've taken a different turn. From the age of five to twenty-three, I survived nine close calls, each one with a brush of death, each one a moment, I could've lost everything.

Why did I make it through, time after time, while Chelsea didn't get that one chance?

This book is my way of honoring her. A collection of near-death stories. Yes, more than that, it's a reminder to cherish life, to protect it, and to understand how fragile it truly is.

2

To the young people who read this:

May these stories wake you up to the reality that life doesn't offer second chances.

Make better choices. Look out for one another. You are not invincible.

Chelsea didn't get a tomorrow. Let's live better because of her.

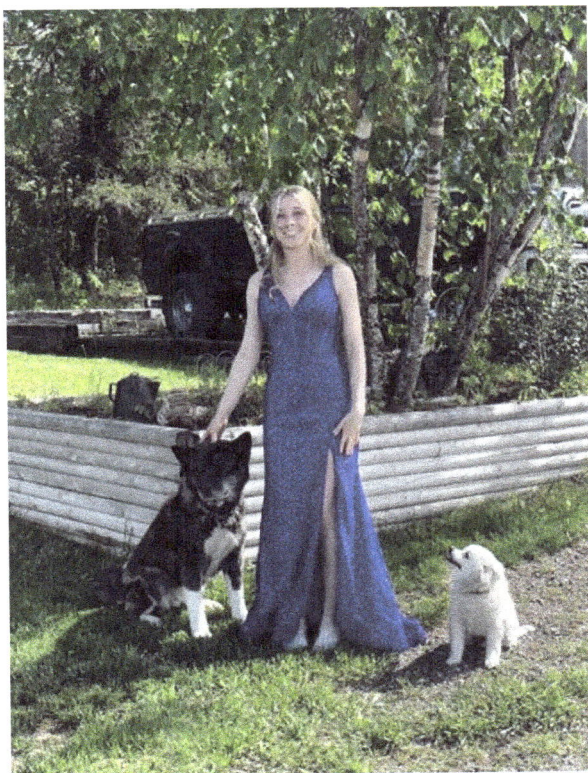

AGE 5

Swimming Incident.

"Off The Deep End"

My sister and I were headed to see our aunt and uncle in Oregon. It was our first trip to the States and our first trip together as brother and sister. So we were both really excited!

The place we stayed at had a huge pool, and both my sister and I were just learning how to swim. My Dad was a very strong swimmer, as he dove and swam a lot when he was in the Navy. After the Navy and meeting my Mom, they were married and moved to Williams Lake and lived there for almost 60 years before they both passed.

My Dad was a big influence on getting both my sister and me to learn to swim quite young...I believe we were around 3? So, after a couple of years and at the prime age of 5, I thought in my small mind that I would be an expert and as strong a swimmer as my Dad.

That was not the case at all, especially that day at the pool in Oregon. Everything that my Dad did, I wanted to emulate and be just like him.

However, there were high mountains to climb and tough tasks to achieve, but I always tried my best and achieved a lot in my younger years. He always told me, "Son... always do your best within reason, but always try to have fun too."

That day at the pool, my sister and I were swimming in the shallow end while my Dad was diving off the deep end and doing his laps.

While watching him, I said to myself, "I want to dive off the deep end."

I got out of the shallow end and told my sister, "I am going to the bathroom."

My Mom wasn't much of a swimmer and she was sitting on a chair poolside. My Dad was doing his many laps, so everyone was busy and didn't notice me during those few minutes.

I walked down to the deep end, tried to dive in with my hands forward...and sploosh! It was more of a belly flop. I basically hit the water and went straight down about 7 feet to the bottom of the pool. My Dad was still swimming, my Mom just looked up at the time I hit the water, and my sister was yelling at my Dad.

I must've been down under for about 30 seconds before my Dad came out, grabbed me, pulled me up, put me on the poolside, and gave me chest pumps to bring me around.

I remember waking up, gasping and spitting water everywhere and heard my mom's screaming and my sister holding me.

AGE 7

Toboggan Fun

"Face First"

The kids in the hood took their toboggans every winter to a steep hill called Water Tower Hill. On one fine and snowy day, things didn't go according to plan.

I was sharing my sled with my neighbor, Karen. I had a crush on her, and I felt it was meant to be that we ride together.

We both got on and decided to strap ourselves in so we could get better momentum sliding down the hill. About halfway down, we caught a rut that threw us off the main run, and we were out of control, sliding very fast down a slippery area.

It got scary because we were headed straight for a big fir tree. At that point, I knew we had to jump, so I unstrapped Karen and pushed her off!

At the very same moment, I looked up, and the huge tree was only a feet away, and I didn't have time to jump. And *smack!* I slammed face-first into that Fir!

I was knocked unconscious and out for at least a minute. Karen and the other kids thought I was dead. Blood was scattered all over the snow.

I finally came to and was bleeding badly from my face, and everyone was screaming!

Karen took her scarf off and wrapped it around my face to slow the bleeding. I will never know how she knew what to do in that situation at the young age of 7.

She helped me walk two blocks to my house and then yelled for help once we got in the basement door.

My mom raced down the stairs and was in a state of shock when she saw me. She grabbed her jacket and rushed me to the hospital. Blood was seeping through the scarf and getting in my eyes and my mouth mixed in with my tears.

The doctor got me into surgery right away. There were cuts all over my face, and I received many stitches!

About a year later, most of the scars disappeared except for one on my chin and one on my eyebrow. It was truly a miracle! That was my first visit to the hospital as a young lad. At the time, I had no idea how many more there were to come!

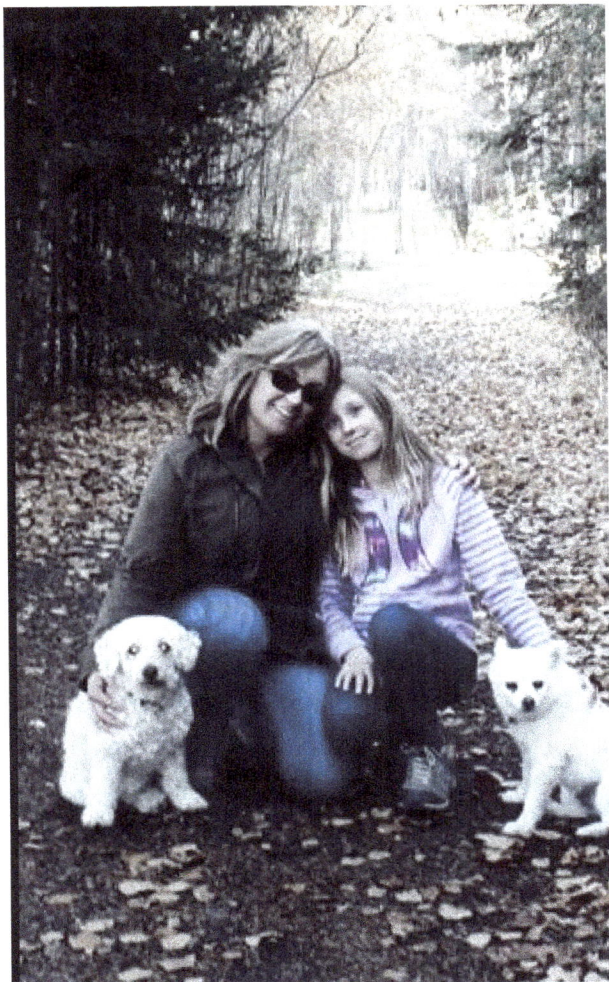

AGE 15

Slalom Water Skiing.

"Showing Off"

It was a beautiful summer day in the middle of July on Chimney Lake, 20 minutes Southwest of our hometown. Many of us kids came in summers there because our parents had cottages on the lake.

Me and my buddies were gearing up for another stellar day on the unusually calm waters. Normally, it was a little wavy, so we all knew that the skiing would be awesome for making sharp cuts. However, it almost led to a tragic crash!

That particular day, we were all trying to outdo each other, typical young lads, and of course, there were a few girls on shore watching us perform.

We were all skiing on one ski, trying to make as sharp of cuts as possible and also trying to touch our elbows on the water without wiping out!

I started my run and felt good, and my Dad was driving the boat. I was going along well, making a few good cuts on either side of the boat, and I think I touched my elbow twice.

Also, near the end of the run, we would let go of the rope about 100 feet shy of the dock, glide in on one ski, and try to sit down gently on the end of the dock. It was all about timing and perfect speed, but most of us could do it without wiping out, and it was a great feeling to finish our run in style.

Unfortunately, that day in question, while showing off to the girls on the shoreline, I waited too late to let go of the rope, and I didn't have time to lean over and dump myself in the lake.

So, I either hit the dock and break both legs or snap one because I was gliding in there around 20 miles per hour, or I lean hard, cover my head and, fly under the dock and hope for the best!

I crashed hard into the logs and rocks and sustained many cuts and bruises, but amazingly, no broken bones or severe injuries!

I lay there covered in blood. Girls were screaming, my buds were freaking out, and my Dad couldn't get there fast enough.

Another miracle and my 2nd trip to the hospital to get stitched up.

Again, very little scarring, mostly to my legs and arms.

AGE 16

Car Accident

"Round, Round We Go"

My best friend, Rob Hinsche (Ginch), was his nickname.

Ginch was a big lad. He stood 6'5" and weighed 240lbs. He was like my elder brother, a gentle giant with a heart of gold.

We just left my folks cottage on Chimney Lake on a late August day. We were driving in Ginch's first vehicle, an older Chevy sedan with lots of power.

Back then, most roads out to the lakes and back country had lots of potholes and they were quite winding too.

We started our trip back home and weren't wearing seat belts at the time.

Back in those days, the seatbelts just went around your waist and many of us didn't wear them too often...

But on that day, since we were cruising along at a good clip and bouncing all over the road, I looked over at Ginch and said, "I think we should put our belts on, and you should slow down a bit."

He looked at me, smiled, and said, buckle up, Scotty!

Moments later, we flew over a cattle guard, blew the front right tire, and then the car flipped and then continued to roll over and over!! Meanwhile, Rob and I were hanging on to the dashboard as tight as we could with our heads down, while the song, "Round, round we go" from the band Trooper was playing on the 8 track.

And then we came to a stop hanging upside down in our seatbelts halfway over a steep embankment.

Thankfully, my parents were only 20 minutes behind us and came upon Rob's totally wrecked vehicle. They helped us out and took us to the hospital with only minor injuries.

Good thing, we put our seatbelts on!

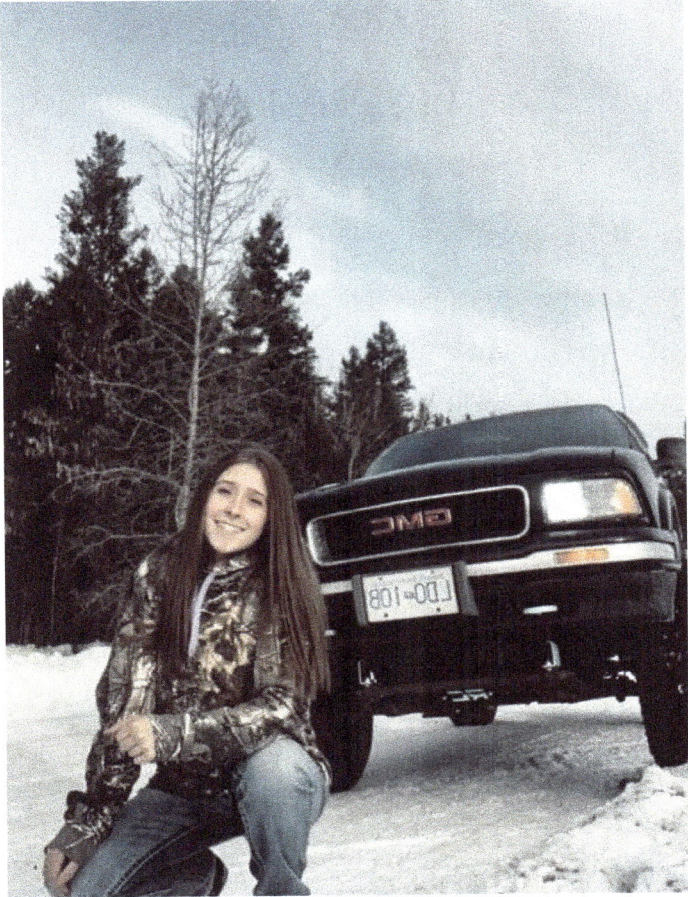

AGE 18

Diving Accident

"Scotty Nipless"

It was mid-May at Chimney Lake again! Lol.

The ice just came off the water a week earlier, and it was time for the annual polar bear dip. My neighbor had this man-made outdoor sauna/steam hut.

A few of us kids who had cottages at Chimney Lake would get together, gather in the outdoor hut, have a couple of drinks...and then dare each other to dive in the freezing cold water.

That day it was a beautiful spring day and quite warm too. There were around 7 or 8 of us, a few gals and a few lads. Two girls went first; they were sisters, and their folks owned the place.

Of course, they wanted to go first to show us boys up.

Now, it was my turn. I started running toward the lake and wanted to make a great jump into the lake.

Not knowing that the water level was down about a foot that year, it was more shallow at the end of the dock. As I flew off the end of the dock, my jump was a little steeper than usual.

When I entered the water, I hit a big log, hitting my chest area. It ripped part of my left nipple off and then continued to bounce off the log and down into a bed of rocks at the bottom of the lake. My hands were over my head, thankfully, so the impact wasn't as bad as it could've been.

However, I hit my chin hard, dislocated my shoulder, and suffered a concussion! I was under the water for around 30 seconds, and there was blood everywhere!

I came up gasping for air in extreme pain, and all the kids were screaming and yelling at me to see if I was okay.

At that time, it was the start of golf season, and I was on the high school golf team getting ready for the provincial championship.

Because of my injuries, especially my shoulder and loss of a nipple, I couldn't think about playing for at least a month. I tried to swing through with the club, but it was too painful!

A few weeks later, I popped into the pro shop to say "hi." The pro at the time, Joe Duffy, who was an old Scotsman who taught me the game, and he was like my second father too, said, "Where the fuck have you been?"

So...I lifted my shirt up, my chest all red and scarred. He looked at me with a strange look and said, "Is that a missing nipple?"

From that day forward, Joe and Assistant Pro, Dan Latin came up with the name Scotty Nipless!

It was kind of like Jack Nicklaus.

That nickname has stayed with me ever since.

It was shortened to Nipper and Nip.

In tournament golf, I write Nip on my ball to identify it.

18

AGE 19

Hockey Injury
"Stick to the throat"

I grew up playing hockey like most Canadian boys and excelled quickly because I was a good skater. I took power skating and figure skating to achieve better balance. This really helped me throughout my young career.

I was playing my first exhibition game of the season for our local junior team. We were playing against the old Kamloops team from the interior of BC, one of the best teams in Canada at the time.

I was still trying to make the team, so I was trying to make an impression on the coaches and scouts. There were two brothers on their team, the Kelly brothers, I think. They were good players but dirty!

I was not a big guy but big enough, and I didn't take any shit from anyone, especially dirty players!

About halfway through the game, we were trailing 6-3, I believe. Our line was on the ice, and my center man skated behind our net to pick up the puck that was left for him by the defenseman.

As he circled around the net, one of the brothers nailed him flat out. As I was skating up the left wing, I just happened to see the hit, did a quick turn, lined the one brother up, and hit him so hard to the boards that the plexiglass came out, and he was slumped over the boards.

I dropped my gloves to fight him, and he declined. As soon as I turned around, he two-handed me with his stick across my throat, and down I went.

I was unconscious for around 2 minutes, I think, and everyone thought I was dead! Meanwhile, a brawl broke out, and there were fights everywhere around me.

My Dad was trying to jump the boards to get at this guy, too. The refs were attending to me and trying to revive me. I finally came around, and I was gasping for air with a huge red welt on my throat.

The paramedics finally arrived and checked me out, and got me to the dressing room. After a while, I started feeling a little better and realized what happened.

At that point, I was so mad that I wanted to go kill this guy, but somehow, I came to my senses and stayed put. After the game, I went up to the coaches and told them I had quit!

They were disappointed because I may have had a promising career...but I knew if it happened again down the road, I probably wouldn't have made it. Who knows?

My Dad was very disappointed because he knew that I had a good chance of making it, so he left for home and didn't give me a ride.

I then decided my hockey career was over and decided to focus on my golf game more seriously the following spring.

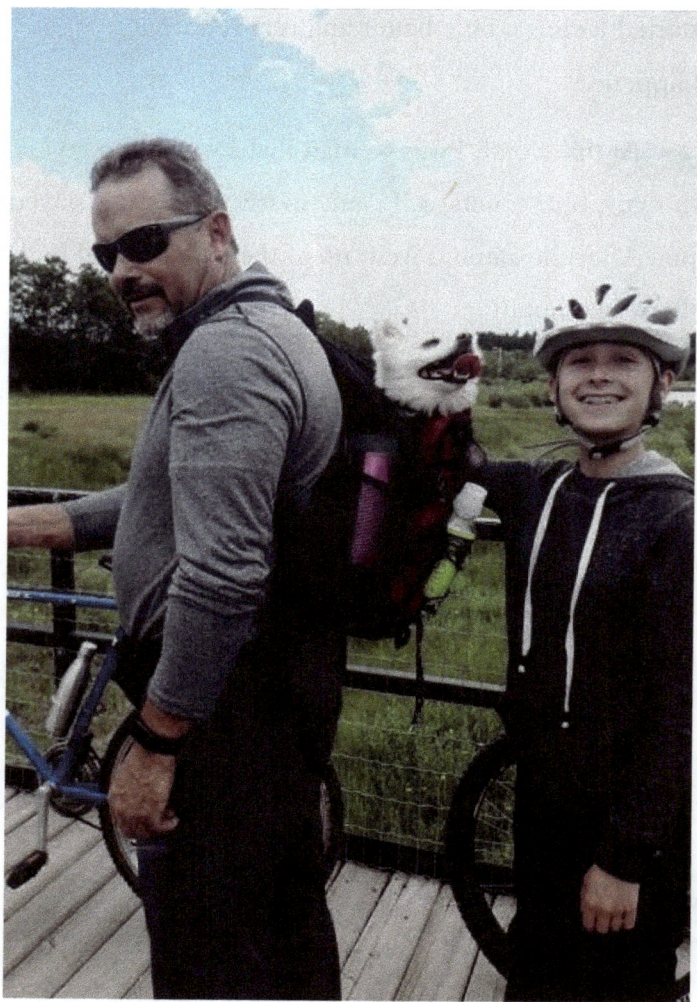

AGE 20

Stampede Open
"Leap of faith"

It was the Stampede Open Golf Tournament.

It is one of the most popular 3-day tournaments in the province.

Good players came from all over B.C. to play and have fun at the Stampede, too. It was always a full field, and the scores were decent. The prizes were good as well, and we even ran a Calcutta and bet on players after the 2nd day. It was well-run, and the food was great too.

I was one of the local favorites, along with a few other guys and our arrogant pro, lol. He was a very good player but not very nice or popular, so he was the guy to beat.

The weather was great that year, and the course was in superb condition.

After day 2, there were about 10 guys close to par, including me, and the pro had a 3-shot lead.

We started the final day, and the battle was on...I birdied four holes on the front and shot 33, and the pro shot 37, so I took a one-shot lead, and the other few guys trailed by 3 to 7 shots.

By #16, I had a 3-shot lead and was getting excited. I said to myself, "I can win this." It was my first win and a big one, too.

Well...I spoke too soon.

I reached the long par 4 -#17 in two and was about 7 feet for birdie. All I had to do was two-putt for par, and I would've sealed the deal.

However, I charged the birdie putt about 6 feet. By then, I started feeling the heat. I got up and lipped out the par putt. I was getting a little mad now, and instead of taking a breath, I went to do the famous quick tap-in and missed my bogey putt. Meanwhile, the pro and a couple of other guys were in the last group watching my collapse and probably couldn't believe what they were watching.

Finally, I tapped in my double bogey, and now, only two shots up on the pro.

I was still mad and trying to settle down a bit, but no! I took my putter and flung it 200 feet out of bounds into the nearby log yard. I then proceeded to run and try to leap over the 4-foot barb-wired fence, and as I was flying through the air, I caught the toe of one foot on the top wire, and it flung me headfirst right into a log!

It stunned me, and I got a big gash on my forehead. Meanwhile, the pro and other players, along with the players on the green, were all yelling at me and worried all at the same time.

I was flaying around, cursing, and trying to find my putter. I found it and put a bandana around my head. My white shirt was soaked in blood and on my shorts and legs too, and I marched over to my bag, picked it up, not saying a word to anyone, and walked over to the 18th tee.

Now, I was sitting on the bench on the 18th tee box in complete silence, and I was shaking and saying to myself, "You can still win."

All I needed was par to win.

I got up, blocked my drive into the woods, and took a smooth triple. I finished tied for 3rd. As I walked up to the green covered in blood, everyone was looking at me in a state of shock.

My folks, my friends, my girlfriend, and the old pro, the Scotsman who taught me the game, all looked at me as if I were some ghost.

I shook hands with everyone, and I was quite embarrassed and disappointed in myself for my actions. Joe, the old pro, walked over. My head was down. He put his hand on my chin, lifted it up, looked into my eyes, and said, "Scott, it's just a game." He then said, "You should take some time away from the game."

I thought he was going to say a couple weeks or the rest of the season, but he said, "I want you to take at least 2 years off and just work on your temperament and short game."

I looked at him with a blank stare, and I realized if I wanted to get to the top of my game, I needed to do what he said.

I then decided to work for a year more and then head off to college.

Two years later, after college, I came back and played my best golf ever for another 7 years. Thank you, Joe!

I got 10 stitches in my head and a concussion from that foolish leap over the fence, and I know it could've been a lot worse!!!

AGE 21

Cuba Month - Keg

"Bad Burn"

A new Keg & Bar Restaurant just opened in Williams Lake, B.C. After one year of being open for business, it was the busiest establishment in town. It was a beautiful cedar structure with a hotel attached to it, and it still stands today.

Often, the management team would host theme months. This particular one was in March, the kick-off to spring! The staff decorated the whole place with crate paper palm trees, streamers, and other decorative objects.

Halfway through March, a bunch of hockey buddies went for dinner and then ended up in the lounge watching hockey and sharing stories and a few jugs of beer. The place was packed with people, well over 200. While we were sitting at the table tipping back a few beers, we also smoked wine-tip cigars. I never smoked, but I did have a cigar once every year or so.

I'm the type of person who talks a lot with his hands, especially after a couple of beers. I was telling a funny story, and accidentally, my right hand with a cigar in it touched the crate paper palm tree. *Poof!* The tree exploded into flames.

I immediately, without hesitation, grabbed the base of the burning tree and started to walk quickly through the lounge to throw outside.

The place was packed, and the structure was all cedar, so the fire would've gone through the building very quickly, and I believe it could've been disastrous!

As I was carrying the burning palm tree through the lounge, I could feel my hand burning, but I couldn't let go because of adrenaline. Also, a piece of the burning tree fell onto my lips and stuck there. I was literally engulfed in flames and could smell burning hair and flesh, but I kept going.

People were throwing jugs of beer, margaritas, and water on me to try and put me out, but very little happened.

I then burst through the doors into the lobby area, and apparently, there was a couple with trench coats checking into the hotel.

They gasped! Quickly took their coats off and threw them onto me. I lay there smoldering and in extreme pain! My buddy came running into the lobby, picked me up, and brought me into the bathroom, and soaked me with water everywhere.

It temporarily relieved some pain, but I knew I was burned badly. He then rushed me to the hospital, and I got into an emergency right away.

I stayed the night and then received the news the next day of my injuries. I couldn't look at myself because I was so scared of what I would look like. I received 3rd degree burns to my right hand and had blisters on my fingers for months. There were 2nd degree burns to my lips, and I had trouble eating food for a while and used lip balm every day for the past 30 years or so. There were mild burns to my face, thankfully, but lost all my eyelashes, eyebrows, and most of my hair on my head.

Amazingly, you can't even tell, and truly, it was a miracle. A few people, doctors too, told me, "We don't know how you survived and with minor burns too." I believe it was my adrenaline and angels watching over me.

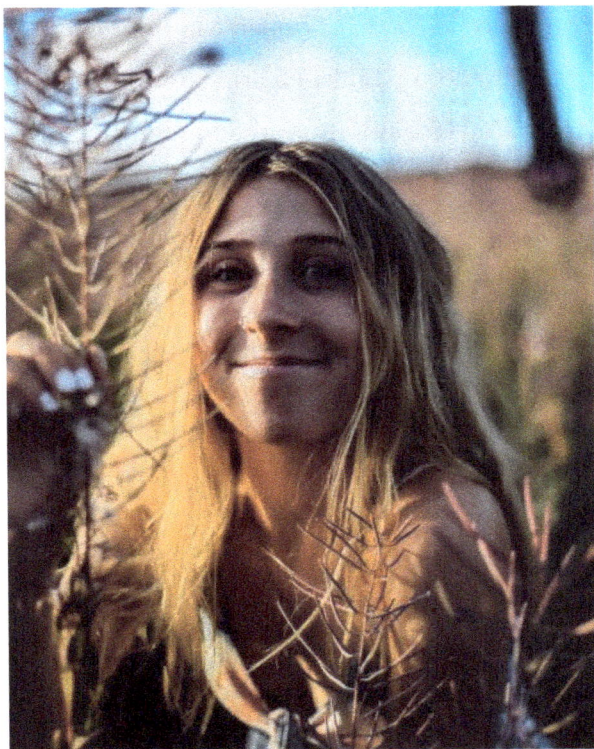

I've seen many great concerts throughout my life, but this one certainly was the most memorable, and I survived it to tell you about it.

AGE 23

Tom Petty and Bob Dylan Concert

"Hey Spike, what do you like?"

When I heard these two icons were coming to Vancouver to perform, I booked four tickets right away for me and my buds. Hearing these two performers sing together would definitely be one of the most memorable highlights of our lives.

The boys and I all got together that day. We went for lunch, had a few beers, and, of course, smoked a bit of whacky tobacco, lol.

I think I have smoked that stuff maybe 10 times in my life.

We arrived about 45 minutes before the concert and got a good place on the floor, not too far from center stage. B.C. Place Stadium was packed with 40,000 people!!

When Petty/Dylan and the band came on the stage, it was the loudest crowd I've ever heard welcoming the two icons to Vancouver.

The cheering and lighters were going full-on!

The concert started, and it was awesome! They were playing all their popular songs, and together, they sounded great.

However, I was hoping they would play "Spike," a song about Tom Petty's dog. It was a very cool song, and I listened to it many times over the years before the concert.

So, I asked my buddy, if I could get up on his shoulders. He was a huge man, 6'5" and 270 lbs, so he could handle my 175 lb frame.

I got up on his shoulders and stood high above all the screaming fans. I started yelling Spike at Petty and Dylan in hopes they might hear me and play the song.

About 30 minutes went by, and no Spike yet.

So, I got down off my buddy's shoulders and thought in my stoned mind that I was going to somehow make them play Spike.

I snuck around behind the stage, very stealth-like, security guards everywhere! Somehow, I managed to sneak up to the stage, grabbed onto the curtain, and started pulling myself up in hopes I could find the center opening in the curtain.

Meanwhile, the crowds were so loud. Security and everyone else were screaming that they didn't even notice what I was doing. I continued scaling the curtain and found the opening. I stuck my head out and started yelling Spike!!! I think I was around 30 feet up off the floor and hanging on for dear life, but I was determined.

All of a sudden, one of the light men turned and shone the light right on my face. The fans were screaming, lighters were flickering, security was shaking the curtain trying to get me down, and then Tom Petty turned and looked at me, said into his Mike in his raspy voice, "Hey son, I think you should get down from there."

The fans were freaking out after that, and I couldn't hang on any longer! I fell off the curtain and thought this is it, 'I'm going to die,' but by a miracle, I landed on the back of a giant man, who I believe saved me from serious injury or potentially death.

I was yelling at them to stop hitting me, and they grabbed me and took me outside. Along the way, I was telling them I just wanted to hear a song and told them I knew that probably wasn't the best approach, but I did get everyone's attention. More importantly, Petty and Dylan's.

A couple of the security guys were laughing, and the other two were quite serious. I kept joking around about the whole episode as they walked me outside.

When we got outside, I asked them if they could leave the door open so that I could listen to the rest of the concert. The security guard convinced the others, and I got to listen to the rest of the concert.

I apologized for my actions, and I told them that I really hoped the security guard who saved my life with his back was going to be okay.

The concert ended, and I waited for my buds outside. By chance, they just happened to walk out the same door that I got escorted out of.

Crazy!!!

They all looked at me in complete amazement, but at the same time, you are crazy, Scotty!!!!!

Another episode of angels watching over me.

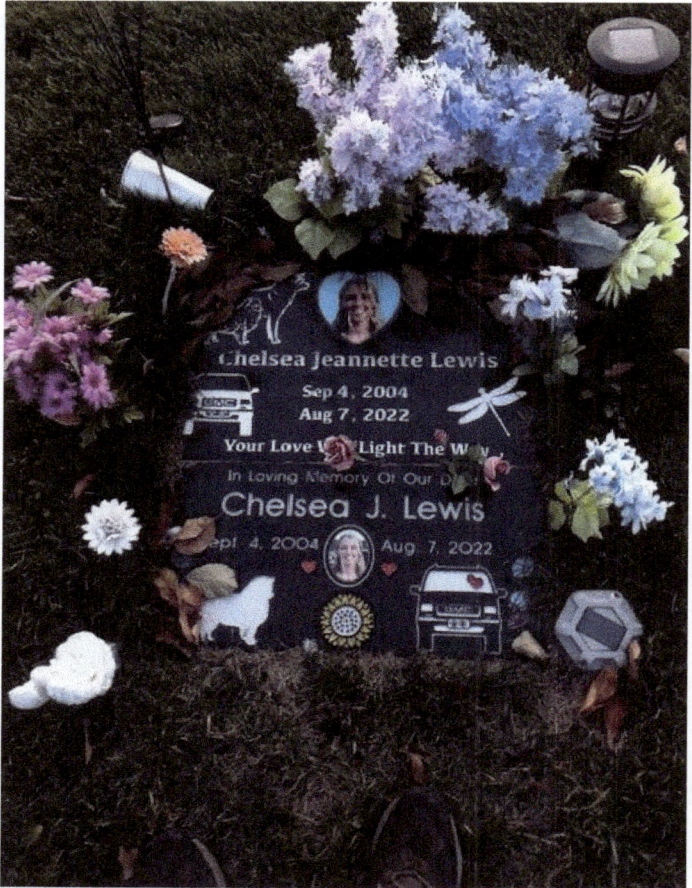